The Better Bath vol. 4: Exfoliating Milk Baths

Written by Lacey Jones

Disclaimer:

The information contained in this book is for general information purposes only.

While we endeavor to keep the information up to date and correct, we make no representations or warranties of any kind, express or implied, about the completeness, accuracy, reliability, suitability or availability with respect to the book or the information, products, services, or related graphics contained in the book for any purpose. Any reliance you place on such information is therefore strictly at your own risk.

None of the information in this this book is meant to be construed as medical advice. It has not been evaluated by the Food and Drug Administration.

Essential oils are powerful compounds. Consult with a medical professional prior to making changes that could impact your health.

Contents

Chapter 1: Introduction to the Better Bath Series of Books

This is the 4th book in the Better Bath Series of books. The first book was on how to make bath bombs, which are little balls that fizz and release fragrances and oils when you toss them in the tub. In the second book, we covered fragranced bath salts that are easy to make and have a number of therapeutic benefits. The 3rd book teaches how to craft sugar scrubs that can be rubbed into the skin to both moisturize and exfoliate it. This is the 4th book in the series and this one's on milk baths.

I'd like to take the time to thank each and every one of my dedicated readers. I wasn't sure what to expect when I started writing these books, and I have to admit the response has been overwhelming.

All of the books in this series are available from Amazon.com and are available as both Kindle and paperback books. If you're new to the series and enjoy this book, I've included links to the other three books in the series in the back of the book. If you're a seasoned Better Bath veteran, thanks for your continued support. I hope you enjoy this book as much and you've enjoyed the previous books in the series.

Chapter 2: What Are Milk Baths?

Aside from water, milk is one of the top beverages consumed when people are thirsty and are looking for refreshment. While there's no doubt milk is a popular beverage, most people don't realize that their favorite beverage is also a great addition to their baths.

The proteins, fats and lactic acid found in milk don't just do your body good on the inside, they can benefit your skin when applied topically as well. A long, luxurious soak in a bath to which milk has been added can provide a number of benefits to your skin, and you'll leave the tub with skin that feels soft and supple. If your skin looks dull and lifeless, a milk bath might be all that's needed to bring it back to life.

It might surprise you to find out this isn't a new fad…Milk baths have been in use for thousands of years. None other than Cleopatra—and a number of other queens and princesses—reportedly used milk baths as part of her beauty routine. Way before the modern skin care creams, salves and lotions that currently populate supermarket shelves were available, men and women who wanted better skin would hop in tub full of milk and soak in it for a while. It wasn't until modern times that milk baths fell out of favor, and they're starting to make a comeback as more and more people return to caring for their skin using natural products.

As milk baths gain in popularity, more and more commercial products are hitting the market. These products provide an easy way for consumers to enjoy the benefits of a milk bath, but they tend to be expensive and often contain synthetic chemicals and preservatives that can be left out when you make your milk baths at home. A look at the label of one popular commercial milk bath reveals it contains sodium laureth sulfate, synthetic fragrances, glycol distearate, EDTA and a number of other chemicals.

I don't know about you, but I'd much rather keep my milk baths natural. When you make your own milk baths at home, you have control over what goes into them, and you can make sure you only include natural ingredients that are beneficial to your skin, skipping the preservatives, synthetic fragrances and surfactants that are unnecessary and may irritate the skin instead of pampering it.

Chapter 3: The Benefits of a Milk Bath

Adding milk to a warm bath can benefit the skin in a number of ways. Here are just some of the many ways a milk bath can be beneficial:

- **The milk exfoliates the skin.** The lactic acid in the milk gently exfoliates the skin, dissolving the dead skin cells sitting at the surface, revealing the healthy skin below.
- **Your skin will feel soft and silky.** The fats and proteins in the milk nourish your skin and leave it feeling silky smooth. I've found this effect to be cumulative. The more milk baths I've got under my belt, the better my skin feels.
- **The milk hydrates and moisturizes the skin.**
- **Milk baths soothe the skin.** If you've got skin conditions that cause redness, rashes and irritation, milk baths can be soothing and may help relieve some of the irritation.
- **You're pampering yourself.** One of the biggest benefits of a milk bath is the relaxation factor. Everyone deserves a little pampering, and a milk bath is a great way to relax and wind down after a long day. Make it even more relaxing by turning on your favorite song and sipping on a cup of hot cocoa (or a glass of wine) while you soak.

While there are a number of skin conditions a milk bath may be able to help eliminate, it's important you check with your health care practitioner prior to attempting to treat anything with milk. Some skin conditions may be worsened by hopping in a tub full of milk, so it's important to double-check prior to using a milk bath.

Chapter 4: The Types of Milk that Can Be Used

When most people think of a milk bath, they think of taking a bath in cow's milk. While cow's milk will definitely work, it isn't the only game in town. There are a number of other varieties of milk that can be used as well.

Animal-based milks are the most popular variety of milk used in milk baths, with the aforementioned cow's milk being the top choice. The milk from other animals can be used as well, with goat, sheep and even buffalo milk being popular choices. The milk from other animals tends to be fattier than cow's milk, which results in the water in the tub feeling creamier and more luxurious. Regardless of the animal it came from, the best type of milk to use is pasteurized whole milk because it contains much of the fat found in raw milk and less of the worry of contamination that's associated with raw milk.

Plant- and nut-based milks can also be used in milk baths. Coconut milk, soy milk, almond milk and rice milk are all popular choices. Just be careful not to use a milk that contains ingredients you're allergic to or you're going to be in for a world of hurt!

Don't be afraid to experiment with the type of milk you use for your milk baths. Your skin will respond differently to the different varieties of milk than other people's skin will respond to them, and you might find one variety works better than the rest. I don't include milk types in most of the recipes because I want you to choose the variety of milk that works best for your skin. Even when milk types are provided, feel free to substitute your favorite type of milk.

Most milk bath recipes call for powdered milk because it's easier to store and will last a lot longer at room temperature than a milk bath made from regular milk. You can store most powdered milk baths at room temperature without having to worry about them going bad before you use them. If you're planning on using your milk bath right away, it can be made with either powdered or liquid milk, or you can even use a can or two of condensed milk.

Chapter 5: Add Fragrance to Your Milk Bath

There's something to be said about simplicity, and you can keep milk baths as simple as you'd like. If you don't feel like mixing and matching ingredients, tossing a cup or two of milk into the tub will exfoliate your skin and leave it feeling great. On the other hand, adding a small handful of ingredients to your milk bath can make the experience even more luxurious by creating a bath that feels great, smells great and carries a number of other properties with it.

If you've read any of my other books, it should come as no surprise that essential oils are one of the key ingredients I like to add to my milk baths to add fragrance to them. If you're new to the series and aren't familiar with essential oils, they're the aromatic essence of plants. They're the compounds found inside of plants that give them their fragrance. If you stop and think of plant you like to smell, there's a pretty good chance that smell can be attributed to essential oils. Now think of a plant you don't like the smell. That's probably due to an essential oil in the plant as well. In addition to smelling great, these oils are packed full of compounds that can provide a number of benefits to the mind, the body and the skin.

While there are literally hundreds of essential oils and oil blends to choose from, be aware that all oils aren't safe for all people. There are some oils that will cause skin irritation and some that are toxic when applied to the skin. There are also some people who will have negative reactions to certain oils that are generally considered safe for most people to use.

The oils I use in the recipes in this book are common oils that are generally considered safe for use, but that doesn't mean they're completely safe for everyone. It's up to the individual to determine which essential oils, if any, are a good match. It's also a good idea to consult with your physician because certain essential oils shouldn't be used when you have medical conditions, are pregnant or you're taking certain medications.

Other ingredients that can be added to milk baths include dried flowers, certain types of tea, salts and sugars. We'll discuss the ingredients that are added to milk baths as we get to them in the recipes section of the book.

Chapter 6: Basic Powdered Milk Bath Recipe

Here's a quick and easy basic recipe you can use to make a powdered milk bath. This recipe can be tailored to suit your individual needs, as the essential oils that are added are entirely up to you. If you don't know what essential oils to add, we'll cover a number of essential oils in future recipes. If you want to try a mild essential oil that's well-tolerated by most people, the Lavender Milk Bath recipe calls for lavender essential oil, which is a good one for most people to start with.

Aside from the essential oils, I only add two ingredients to the basic milk bath recipe. I add baking soda, which acts as a water softener and helps soften the skin, and I add cornstarch, which is added because it's soothing to the skin and adds volume to the recipe.

Ingredients:

4 cups powdered milk
1 cup baking soda
1 cup cornstarch
20 to 25 drops of your favorite essential oil

Directions:

1. Combine all of the dry ingredients in a container.
2. Place the lid onto the container and shake it until all of the ingredients are thoroughly mixed.

3. Add the essential oil to the container.
4. Shake the container again to disperse the essential oil throughout the milk bath.
5. Store the milk bath in an airtight container in a cool, dry place until you're ready to use it.
6. To use the milk bath, add a cup or two of it to your bathtub while the water is still running. Sit down and soak for a while, taking in the fragrance of the essential oils.

Chapter 7: Whole Milk Bath

This milk bath is the same as the previous milk bath, but it calls for liquid milk instead of powdered milk. This recipe is best when used within a day or two of being made. If you want to store it, keep it in the fridge, and make sure you use it before the milk turns. You don't want to take a sour milk bath!

As far as benefits go, you get pretty much the same effect with this recipe as you do when powdered milk is used. The main difference between the two is the ease of storage when powdered milk is used.

Ingredients:

4 cups whole milk
1 cup baking soda
1 cup cornstarch
20 to 25 drops of your favorite essential oil

Directions:

1. Combine all of the ingredients except the essential oil in a container.
2. Place the lid onto the container and shake it until all of the ingredients are thoroughly mixed.
3. Add the essential oil to the container.
4. Shake the container again to disperse the essential oil throughout the milk bath.
5. Store the milk bath in an airtight container in a cool, dry place until you're ready to use it.

6. To use the milk bath, add a cup or two of it to your bathtub while the water is still running. Sit down and soak for a while, taking in the fragrance of the essential oils.

Chapter 8: Almond Milk Bath

I used liquid almond milk in this recipe because, to my knowledge, powdered almond milk doesn't exist. It worked out to the benefit of the recipe because it allowed me to add another liquid ingredient that's full of creamy, luxurious fats. The coconut cream added to this recipe takes things to a whole new level of luxury.

This recipe doesn't contain any animal fats, so it's a good choice for those who are opposed to using animal milk. Fragrance is up to you. You can use your favorite essential oil or essential oil blend.

Ingredients:

2 cups almond milk
½ cup coconut cream
½ cup baking soda
½ cup cornstarch
10 to 15 drops of your favorite essential oil

Directions:

1. Combine all of the ingredients except the essential oil in a container.
2. Place the lid onto the container and shake it until all of the ingredients are thoroughly mixed.
3. Add the essential oil to the container.
4. Shake the container again to disperse the essential oil throughout the milk bath.

5. Do not attempt to store this recipe for more than a day or two. If you do store it, keep it in the fridge. To use the milk bath, add a cup or two of it to your bathtub while the water is still running. Sit down and soak for a while, taking in the fragrance of the essential oils.

Chapter 9: Lavender Milk Bath

If you're new to the world of essential oils, lavender essential oil is a great jumping off point because it falls on the milder end of the spectrum as far as the potential for irritation is concerned. While there are a select few people who can't tolerate lavender essential oil, most individuals can use it without a problem, and it's the number one most-popular essential oil in existence.

Lavender essential oil has healing properties that make it a great choice for dry, weathered skin. It's a soothing, calming oil that will help knock out inflammation and is used as a home remedy for a number of skin conditions. It can also be used on minor cuts, burns and scrapes to promote faster healing and prevent infection.

When you soak in a tub with lavender oil added, you don't just soothe your skin with the oil. The fragrance is calming, and you'll leave the tub feeling relaxed. Lavender milk baths are best when used in the evening because you'll probably be ready for bed once you're done soaking in the tub.

Basic Lavender Milk Bath

This basic lavender milk bath is a decent one to use on its own if you want something simple that has lavender essential oil in it.

It's also a good jumping-off point for working on oil blends that combine lavender essential oil with other essential oils to create fragrant blends that combine the benefits of the oils in the blend. Lavender essential oil is one of the best oils for blending because it melds well with most other essential oils.

Ingredients:

4 cups powdered milk
1 cup baking soda
1 cup cornstarch
20 to 30 drops of lavender essential oil

Directions:

1. Combine all of the ingredients except the lavender essential oil in a container.
2. Place the lid onto the container and shake it until all of the ingredients are thoroughly mixed.
3. Add the lavender essential oil to the container.
4. Shake the container again to disperse the essential oil throughout the milk bath.
5. Store the milk bath in an airtight container in a cool, dry place until you're ready to use it.
6. To use the milk bath, add a cup or two of it to your bathtub while the water is still running. Sit down and

soak for a while, taking in the fragrance of the essential oils.

Dried Lavender Milk Bath

The basic lavender milk bath is a good recipe to use at home when you aren't worried about aesthetic value and just want to soak in a tub that smell like lavender and gives you all the benefits of lavender essential oil. The downside is it's rather plain looking and doesn't make for a great gift. This recipe adds a cup of crumbled dried lavender flowers to the previous recipe to create a milk bath that's functionally the same as the previous one, but is a better gift because it looks more complex.

Make sure you crumble the dried lavender into small pieces or you run the risk of clogging your drain with dried lavender.

Ingredients:

4 cups powdered milk
1 cup baking soda
1 cup cornstarch
2 to 3 dried lavender sprigs
20 to 30 drops of lavender essential oil

Directions:

1. Crumble the dried lavender sprigs.
2. Combine all of the ingredients except the lavender essential oil in a container.
3. Place the lid onto the container and shake it until all of the ingredients are thoroughly mixed.
4. Add the lavender essential oil to the container.

5. Shake the container again to disperse the essential oil throughout the milk bath.
6. Store the milk bath in an airtight container in a cool, dry place until you're ready to use it.
7. To use the milk bath, add a cup or two of it to your bathtub while the water is still running.

Lavender Honey Milk Bath

It's amazing what a difference the addition of a single ingredient can make. Add honey to a lavender milk bath and you'll end up with a sweet-smelling milk bath that leaves your skin feeling healthy and silky-smooth. Don't worry about getting out of the tub feeling sticky. The honey dissolves in the warm water and doesn't leave a residue behind on your skin.

This recipe calls for liquid milk because it's difficult to get the honey to properly mix into powdered milk without causing the milk to clump up.

Ingredients:

2 cups whole milk
½ cup baking soda
½ cup cornstarch
2 to 3 dried lavender sprigs
¼ cup raw honey
10 to 20 drops of lavender essential oil

Directions:

1. Crumble the dried lavender sprigs.
2. Combine all of the ingredients except the lavender essential oil in a container.
3. Place the lid onto the container and shake it until all of the ingredients are thoroughly mixed.
4. Add the lavender essential oil to the container.
5. Shake the container again to disperse the essential oil throughout the milk bath.

6. This recipe doesn't store well and is best when used immediately after making it. An alternate solution is to make a lavender milk bath using powdered milk and add the honey to the tub when you add the milk bath.

7. To use the milk bath, add a cup or two of it to your bathtub while the water is still running.

Lavender Chamomile Milk Bath

There are two basic types of chamomile that are commonly used in skin care products: Roman chamomile and German chamomile. Both varieties of chamomile are strongly anti-inflammatory and contain a number of compounds that are considered beneficial to the skin. I prefer Roman chamomile to German chamomile because it has a sweet fragrance that has hints of apple to it.

This recipe doubles up on the chamomile by adding chamomile tea to the recipe as well. If you don't want to deal with the crumbled tea leaves in the bath, you can place the milk bath into a thin mesh baggy and toss the baggy into the tub.

Ingredients:

4 cups powdered milk
1 cup baking soda
1 cup cornstarch
2 tablespoons dried chamomile tea
20 drops of Roman chamomile essential oil

Directions:

1. Crumble the chamomile tea. Make sure the tea leaves are broken into small pieces. If you don't have loose-leaf tea available, you can open a couple chamomile tea bags and use the tea inside.
2. Combine all of the ingredients except the Roman chamomile essential oil in a container.

3. Place the lid onto the container and shake it until all of the ingredients are thoroughly mixed.
4. Add the Roman chamomile essential oil to the container.
5. Shake the container again to disperse the essential oil throughout the milk bath.
6. Store the milk bath in an airtight container in a cool, dry place until you're ready to use it.
7. To use the milk bath, add a cup or two of it to your bathtub while the water is still running. Let it sit for 10 minutes before climbing in, so the tea has time to steep.

Lavender Oat Bath

Here's another take on the basic lavender milk bath. This one adds ground oatmeal to the mix.

While bathing in an oatmeal bath might seem strange, the oatmeal quickly disperses into the bath water, creating a creamy, luxurious bath that you aren't going to want to get out of. The key to getting this one right is to make sure the oatmeal is properly ground. You don't want any whole oats floating around that are going to stick to you when you get out of the bath.

This recipe calls for your basic lavender essential oil, but it'll work with pretty much any of the other recipes in the book. All you have to do is add a cup of ground oatmeal to the recipe and stir it in.

Ingredients:

4 cups powdered milk
1 cup baking soda
1 cup cornstarch
1 cup oatmeal
15 to 20 drops lavender essential oil

Directions:

1. Grind the cup of oatmeal. You can do this in a food processor, a blender or a spice grinder. The key is grind it until it's broken up into small pieces.
2. Combine all of the ingredients except the lavender essential oil in a container.

3. Place the lid onto the container and shake it until all of the ingredients are thoroughly mixed.
4. Add the lavender essential oil to the container.
5. Shake the container again to disperse the essential oil throughout the milk bath.
6. Store the milk bath in an airtight container in a cool, dry place until you're ready to use it.
7. To use the milk bath, add a cup or two of it to your bathtub while the water is still running. Let it sit for 10 minutes to give the oatmeal time to disperse into the bath water.

Chapter 10: Tea Tree Milk Bath

There are a growing number of people who swear by tea tree essential oil and use it for a number of hygienic and home remedy purposes. I've heard of people using it for everything from insect bites to acne to healing up cuts and wounds. It's got regenerative and healing properties and is a great oil to add to the bath when you have skin that's cracked and dry or is damaged.

The key is to make sure you don't add too much tea tree oil to your products. A little bit of tea tree oil goes a long way, and you don't want to add too much or you might find the bath ends up being rather uncomfortable. I've heard complaints from people who used too much tea tree oil who said their legs and arms started itching and burning after a short soak in the tub. When I asked one of the people how much tea tree oil they'd used, they said they'd added an entire teaspoon of oil to the tub. That's way too much oil, when you consider most recipes only call for 10 to 20 drops of oil being added to the entire recipe.

Of course, there's always the potential for irritation, as is the case with any essential oil, so start with a small amount and test it to make sure your skin is able to tolerate it.

Tea Tree Milk Bath Recipe

Ingredients:

4 cups powdered milk
1 cup baking soda
1 cup cornstarch
10 to 15 drops tea tree essential oil

Directions:

1. Combine all of the ingredients except the tea tree essential oil in a container.
2. Place the lid onto the container and shake it until all of the ingredients are thoroughly mixed.
3. Add the tea tree essential oil to the container.
4. Shake the container again to disperse the essential oil throughout the milk bath.
5. Store the milk bath in an airtight container in a cool, dry place until you're ready to use it.

Chapter 11: Mint Milk Baths

Peppermint essential oil is another oil that's considered a good oil for skin care. It's used to provide relief to unhealthy and damaged skin and it might even ease muscle and joint pain and itching. It's a cooling oil that opens up the capillaries in the areas it comes in contact with, creating a sensation similar to that of vapor rub.

In addition to being beneficial to the skin, peppermint essential oil has stimulant properties that will leave you feeling awake and rejuvenated. Mint milk baths are best when used in the mornings, as opposed to the evenings, because of their stimulant properties. If you've got a long day ahead of you, a mint-infused milk bath may be just what you need to make it through the day. If you're trying to wind down and put a long day behind you, steer clear of mint milk baths.

Peppermint essential oil is one of the more powerful oils you're going to see used in recipes in this book, and not everyone is able to tolerate it. Test it by diluting a small amount of peppermint oil with coconut oil and applying it to a small patch of skin. Wait 24 hours to see if redness or a rash develops. If you see redness or a rash, discontinue use of peppermint oil and try other less intense oils.

Peppermint Milk Bath Recipe

Ingredients:

4 cups powdered milk
1 cup baking soda
1 cup cornstarch
10 to 15 drops peppermint essential oil

Directions:

1. Combine all of the ingredients except the peppermint essential oil in a container.
2. Place the lid onto the container and shake it until all of the ingredients are thoroughly mixed.
3. Add the peppermint essential oil to the container.
4. Shake the container again to disperse the essential oil throughout the milk bath.
5. Store the milk bath in an airtight container in a cool, dry place until you're ready to use it.

Rosemary Mint Milk Bath

Rosemary essential oil is taken from the culinary herb and smells like a concentrated version of the rosemary you're probably already familiar with. It's said to carry a number of benefits, including being analgesic, antibacterial and anti-inflammatory. It works well to provide relief from a number of skin conditions and is a stimulant oil that will leave you feeling awake and aware just like peppermint oil.

The combination of peppermint essential oil and rosemary essential oil in this recipe is a powerful one and may not be a good choice for those who have sensitive skin. If you can't tolerate peppermint essential oil on its own, don't even think about trying this recipe.

Ingredients:

4 cups powdered milk
1 cup baking soda
1 cup cornstarch
5 to 10 drops peppermint essential oil
5 to 10 drops rosemary essential oil

Directions:

1. Combine all of the ingredients except the peppermint and rosemary essential oils in a container.
2. Place the lid onto the container and shake it until all of the ingredients are thoroughly mixed.
3. Add the peppermint and rosemary essential oil to the container.

4. Shake the container again to disperse the essential oils throughout the milk bath.
5. Store the milk bath in an airtight container in a cool, dry place until you're ready to use it.

Mild Minty Milk Bath

If you're looking for something that isn't quite as intense as the previous recipe, you might enjoy this recipe a little more. It swaps the peppermint essential oil, which is pretty powerful, for a couple tablespoons of dried peppermint leaves, which aren't quite as strong. You'll still get a minty fragrance and some of the benefits of peppermint oil, but you won't get as much of the cooling sensation.

Ingredients:

4 cups powdered milk
1 cup baking soda
1 cup cornstarch
2 tablespoons dried peppermint leaves, crumbled

Directions:

1. Crumble the peppermint leaves into small pieces.
2. Add all of the ingredients to a container.
3. Place the lid onto the container and shake it until all of the ingredients are thoroughly mixed.
4. Store the milk bath in an airtight container in a cool, dry place until you're ready to use it.
5. Let this recipe steep for a while in the tub before you climb in to give the peppermint leaves time to do their thing.

Hot Chocolate Mint Bath

If you've ever wondered what it would be like to be a marshmallow floating around in a glass of hot chocolate, this recipe is about as close as you're going to get. OK, I know I'm not the only one who has thought about this, am I? The best part is the cocoa powder used in this recipe is actually beneficial to the skin. It's packed clear full of antioxidant compounds that will help eliminate the free radicals that cause all sorts of problems with the skin.

Ingredients:

4 cups powdered milk
1 cup baking soda
1 cup cornstarch
½ cup unsweetened cocoa powder
10 to 15 drops peppermint essential oil

Directions:

1. Combine all of the ingredients except the peppermint essential oil in a container.
2. Place the lid onto the container and shake it until all of the ingredients are thoroughly mixed.
3. Add the peppermint essential oil to the container.
4. Shake the container again to disperse the essential oil throughout the milk bath.
5. Store the milk bath in an airtight container in a cool, dry place until you're ready to use it.

Eucalyptus Mint Cold Buster Milk Bath

If you've got a cold and are looking for some relief from the coughing and congestion, this eucalyptus mint milk bath might help clear your head up a bit. The combination of these two oils is a potent one that might be powerful enough to help your respiratory system get back on track.

Peppermint and eucalyptus essential oil are powerful oils on their own and are even more powerful when combined, so this recipe isn't for those with sensitive skin. Even if you're able to tolerate it, a short soak while you breathe deeply is all that's needed.

Ingredients:

4 cups powdered milk
1 cup baking soda
1 cup cornstarch
10 drops eucalyptus essential oil
10 to 15 drops peppermint essential oil

Directions:

1. Combine all of the ingredients except the peppermint and eucalyptus essential oils in a container.
2. Place the lid onto the container and shake it until all of the ingredients are thoroughly mixed.
3. Add the peppermint and eucalyptus essential oils to the container.
4. Shake the container again to disperse the essential oil throughout the milk bath.

5. Store the milk bath in an airtight container in a cool, dry place until you're ready to use it.

Chapter 12: Touch of Rose

If you like the fragrance of roses, you're going to love this recipe. It's a well-known fact that Cleopatra and a number of other queens and princesses indulged in milk baths. When I soak in a tub to which I've added my touch of rose milk bath to, I close my eyes and almost feel like a beautiful princess soaking in a lavish tub filled with milk and rose petals.

The rose essential oil this recipe calls for is rather expensive. It's a great-smelling oil that is beneficial to the skin, but be prepared for sticker shock when you go to add it to your cart. The reason it costs so much is because rose essential oil has to be taken from the petals of roses and it takes a lot of roses to get just a tiny amount of essential oil. The good news is you're only going to be using 15 to 20 drops at a time, so a small bottle will last quite some time.

Touch of Rose Recipe

Ingredients:

4 cups powdered milk
1 cup baking soda
1 cup cornstarch
½ cup dried rose petals
15 to 20 drops of rose essential oil

Directions:

1. Crumble the dried rose petals into tiny pieces.
2. Combine all of the ingredients except the rose essential oil in a container.
3. Place the lid onto the container and shake it until all of the ingredients are thoroughly mixed.
4. Add the essential oil to the container.
5. Shake the container again to disperse the essential oil throughout the milk bath.
6. Store the milk bath in an airtight container in a cool, dry place until you're ready to use it.

Alternative Touch of Rose Recipe

If you want to take a bath that smells like roses, but don't want to pay the price being asked for rose essential oil, this recipe is a good alternative. It uses rose geranium essential oil, which doesn't exactly smell like roses, but is close enough that most people can't tell the difference. The two oils have similar enough properties to where you won't lose too much by making the switch.

Ingredients:

4 cups powdered milk
1 cup baking soda
1 cup cornstarch
½ cup dried rose petals
20 to 25 drops of rose geranium essential oil

Directions:

1. Crumble the dried rose petals into tiny pieces.
2. Combine all of the ingredients except the rose geranium essential oil in a container.
3. Place the lid onto the container and shake it until all of the ingredients are thoroughly mixed.
4. Add the essential oil to the container.
5. Shake the container again to disperse the essential oil throughout the milk bath.
6. Store the milk bath in an airtight container in a cool, dry place until you're ready to use it.

Chapter 13: Peaches and Cream

I suppose you could make this milk bath with powdered milk and use dried peach tea and it would be passable, but I'm a big fan of the creaminess the whole milk adds to the bath. If you want your bath to be peachier, you can blend a ripe peach up and add it to the bath, but I didn't care for the little peach particle that got *everywhere*.

I've seen recipes online for peaches and cream milk baths that call for peach essential oil, which doesn't exist. There are a few manufacturers selling what they claim is peach essential oil, and I strongly suspect it's some sort of synthetic blend or maybe a combination of things made to smell like peaches.

Peaches and Cream Recipe

Ingredients:

2 cups whole milk
½ cup baking soda
½ cup cornstarch
1 cup peach tea

Directions:

1. Brew the peach tea as strong as you can get it.
2. Combine all of the ingredients in a container.
3. Place the lid onto the container and shake it until all of the ingredients are thoroughly mixed.

4. Do not attempt to store this recipe. Use it shortly after making it for best results.

Chapter 14: Milk and Tea

This recipe is one that's open for interpretation, as you can use pretty much any of your favorite teas for drinking to add fragrance and antioxidant power to your milk bath. I've used green tea, chamomile tea, and the previous recipe called for peach tea.

Depending on the type of tea used, you may or may not want to add essential oils for a bit of extra fragrance.

Milk and Tea Recipe

Ingredients:

4 cups powdered milk
½ cup baking soda
½ cup cornstarch
2 to 4 tablespoons of your favorite tea
OPTIONAL: 10 to 15 drops of your favorite essential oil or essential oil blend.

Directions:

1. Crumble the tea leaves into fine pieces. You want them broken up as small as you can get them if you're going to be tossing the milk bath directly into the tub.
2. Combine all of the ingredients in a container.
3. Place the lid onto the container and shake it until all of the ingredients are thoroughly mixed.

4. If you're adding essential oils to the recipe, add them at this time and shake the container until they're mixed in.
5. Store this recipe in an airtight container until you're ready to use it.

Previous Books in the Series

If you're new to the Better Bath series and want the other two books, they're available from Amazon.com. The first book is about bath bombs and is available here:

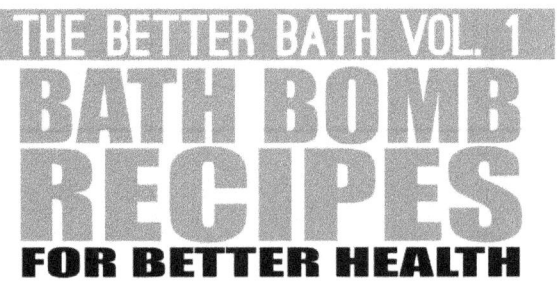

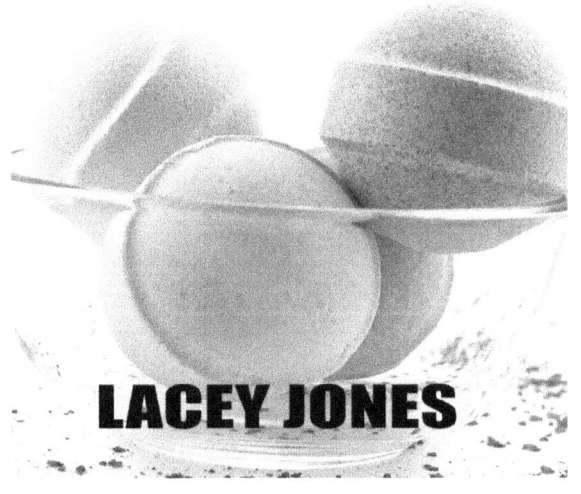

http://www.amazon.com/Bath-Bomb-Recipes-Better-Health-ebook/dp/B00RKJ2854/

The second book in the series teaches you how to make fragranced bath salts. You can purchase that book here:

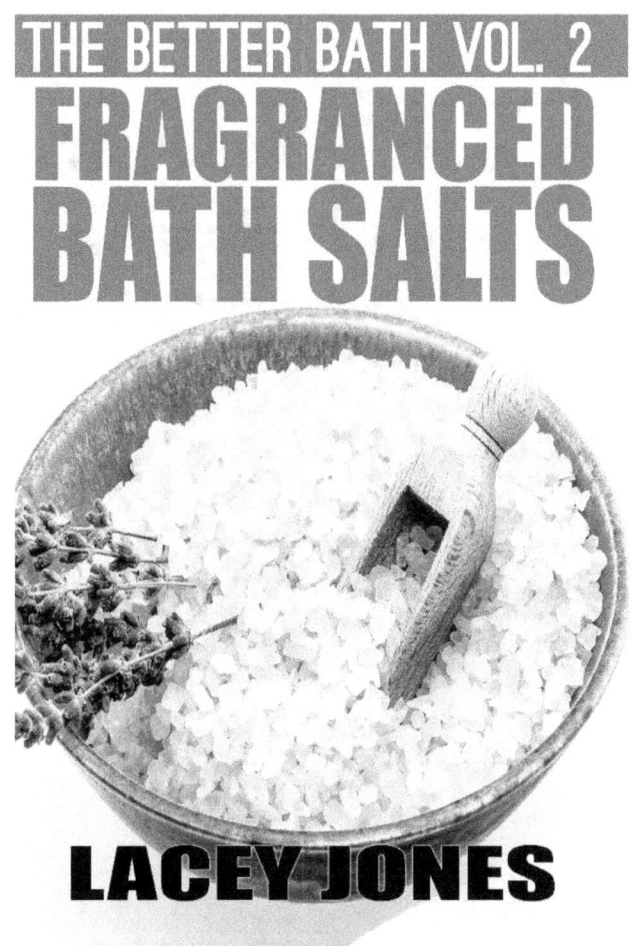

http://www.amazon.com/Better-Bath-vol-Fragranced-Salts-ebook/dp/B00ROX75Q8

The third book in the series is on making amazing sugar scrubs that can be used to exfoliate your skin:

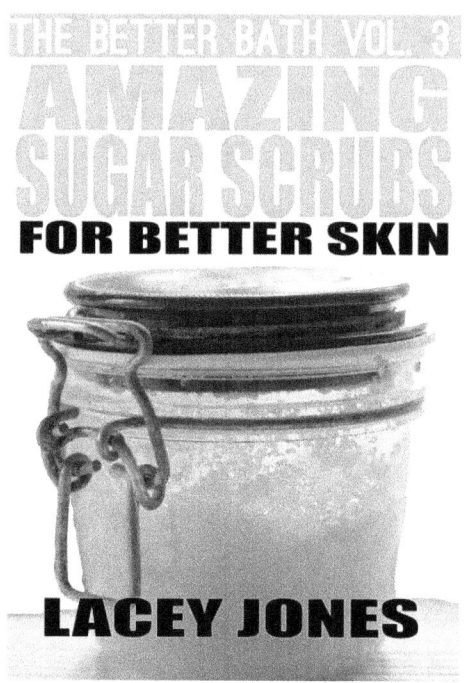

http://www.amazon.com/dp/B00SHR7AP6

www.ingramcontent.com/pod-product-compliance
Lightning Source LLC
Chambersburg PA
CBHW071136280526
45787CB00003B/1304